APPLYING SMART TECHNOLOGY TO VALUE-BASED CARE

The Future of Healthcare is Now

Tom Scaletta, MD

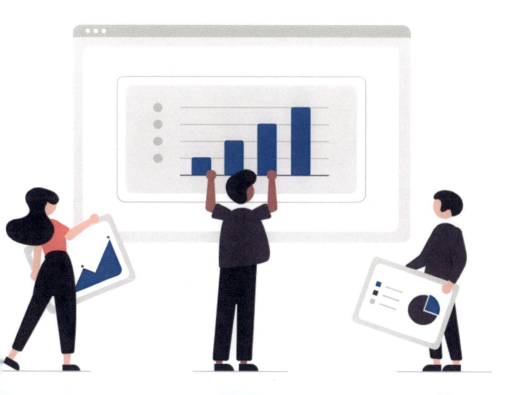

Table of Contents

Origin of Artificial Intelligence 5

Smart Technology 9

Automation 10

Artificial Intelligence 12

Machine Learning 13

    Generative AI 19

    Large Language Models 20

    ChatGPT 21

    Natural Language Processing/Speech Recognition 23

    Predictive Analytics 24

Value-Based Care 26

    Transition from Fee-for-Service 26

    Frameworks 28

    Quality 29

    Utilization 30

    Efficiency 30

    Satisfaction 31

    Teamwork 31

    QUEST Dependencies 32

Coupling AI and VBC 34
Integration 34
Quality Focus 34
Utilization Focus 35
Efficiency Focus 36
Satisfaction Focus 37
Teamwork Focus 38

AI Across the VBC Continuum 39
Overview 39
Pre-Acute Care 40
Acute Care 40
Post-Acute Care 41
End-of-Life Care 42

Case Management 43
Emergency Department 43
Inpatient 43
Post-Hospitalization 44

Patient-Centeredness 45
Personalized Care 45
AI and Empathy 46
Patient Activation 48

AI Risks and Challenges	49
Change Management	52
Simon Sinek: Start With Why	52
BJ Fogg: Change Driver	53
Knoster's Model for Managing Change	54
Everett M Rogers: The Diffusion of Innovation	55
AI Ethics and Bias	57
Summary	58
Case Studies	59
Hospitalization Avoidance	59
ED Overuse Reduction	63

Origin of Artificial Intelligence

Artificial intelligence (AI) is the ability of a computer to complete human tasks, allowing a machine to exceed human knowledge and replace human workflows. Alan Turing is credited with describing the concept in 1950, and John McCarthy coined the term AI in 1955. Chatbots and humanoid robots appeared in the 1960s. Often referred to as the "AI winter," advancements in the field were idle for 45 years since data storage systems and computer processing speeds were inadequate.

- 1950 (Turing)
- 1955 (McCarthy)
- 1964 (Chatbot)
- 1966 (Robot)

- 2011 (Siri)
- 2012 (Deep Learning)
- 2014 (Alexa)
- 2021 (ChatGPT)

45-year Winter awaiting space/speed

Stanley Kubrick's 1968 film, "2001: A Space Odyssey,"[1] forecasted the future, portraying a tense dialogue between astronaut Dave Bowman and HAL, shorthand

---

1 - https://en.wikipedia.org/wiki/2001:_A_Space_Odyssey

for his Heuristically-programmed ALgorithmic computer. *Heuristics* is a term for mental shortcuts used to make fast decisions and solve problems.

On their mission to Jupiter, HAL initiates a lethal sequence that claims the lives of the ship's crew members. The following exchange transpires when Dave tries to shut down HAL.

*DAVE: Open the pod bay doors, Hal.
HAL: I'm sorry, Dave. I'm afraid I can't do that.
DAVE: What's the problem?
HAL: I think you know what the problem is just as well as I do.
DAVE: What are you talking about, Hal?
HAL: This mission is too important for me to allow you to jeopardize it.*

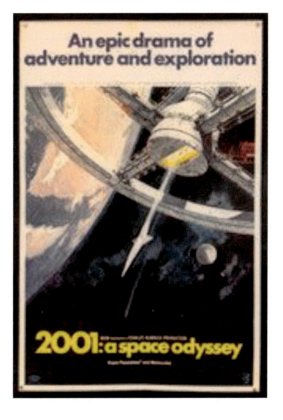

This handbook outlines two significant and simultaneous developments in the healthcare sector: smart technology and value-based care (VBC). In 2023, a pivotal shift occurred as Medicare Advantage enrollees surpassed those in traditional Medicare. [2] This event marked a transition from fee-for-service (FFS) to VBC, which most healthcare payers are adopting.

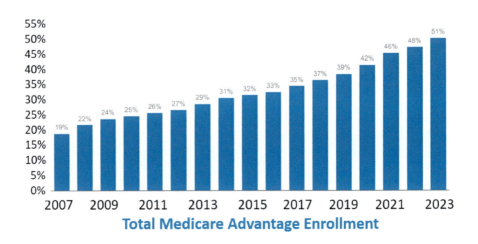

Total Medicare Advantage Enrollment

The CMS Innovation Center, created by Congress in 2010, seeks to enhance healthcare quality while mitigating costs. It intends to expedite the transition from a volume-based to a value-based payment model.

---

2 - https://en.wikipedia.org/wiki/2001:_A_Space_Odyssey

In 2023, it introduced five objectives to ensure access to a health system that achieves high-quality, affordable, person-centered care for all Americans.

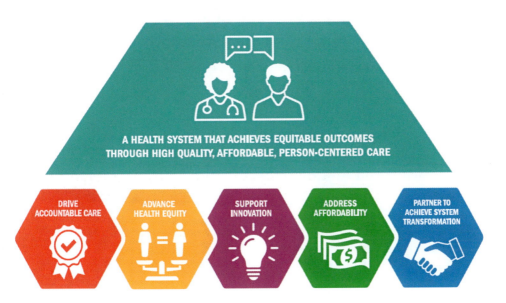

Additionally, there has been an exponential surge in the integration of automation and artificial intelligence applications throughout the spectrum of patient care needs. This handbook uses the QUEST framework to explore the dynamic intersection of smart technology and VBC, encompassing quality, utilization, efficiency, satisfaction, and teamwork.

Smart Technology

Smart technology refers to computer programs and smartphone applications that utilize automation and artificial intelligence to simplify workflows, improve performance, and achieve business goals. What makes smart technology "smart" is its ability to adapt to change.

Smart technology includes automation and AI. The most sophisticated AI tools involve "deep learning," a subset of machine learning.

AI Hierarchy

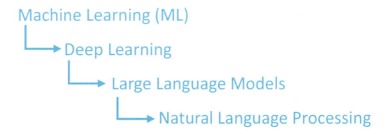

Automation

Automation involves using technology to execute repetitive tasks based on predefined rules without human intervention. [3] Decision trees are structured to choose between multiple options based on conditions (inputs), leading to an optimal decision (output).

The first medical rules-based expert system, Mycin, was developed at Stanford University by Bruce Buchanan and Edward Shortliffe in the 1970s. It helped diagnose infections by cross-referencing patient symptoms with a database. The program generated clarifying branch questions and ranked potential diagnoses based on severity and likelihood, offering treatment recommendations.

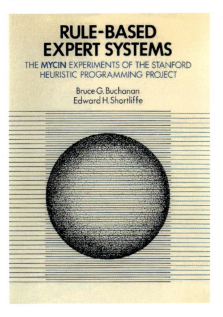

Workflow automation enhances operational efficiency, accuracy, and agility while enabling teams to focus on

---

3 - https://en.wikipedia.org/wiki/Weak_artificial_intelligence

more creative and critical jobs. Though automation simplifies tasks, its creation is complex. A comprehensive understanding of workflows, pain points, and task suitability are prerequisites to success. Program design entails logical sequences, decision points, and governing rules. Data security and unbiased results are imperative in healthcare. Rigorous testing and user training ensure that AI systems function as intended. Continuous monitoring is necessary to maintain peak performance, accuracy, and efficiency.

In the past, healthcare providers relied on manual methods, such as telephone calls or paper-based appointment reminder cards. This process was time-consuming, error-prone, and often resulted in many missed appointments.

An example of automation in healthcare is SMS-based appointment reminders, which engage patients, reduce no-show rates, and improve care.

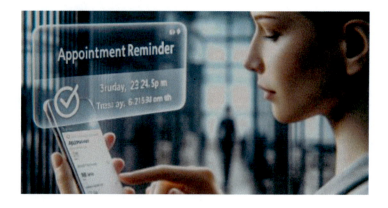

Artificial Intelligence

AI is the science of designing computer systems to emulate human cognition. AI systems process data, create fundamental insights, tackle specific tasks, and streamline human workflows.

AI is a means of transforming unstructured data into structured formats. This task is facilitated by mining vast databases, discerning intricate patterns, and making intelligent recommendations.

"Super AI" is a conceptual realm where machines outperform humans across all tasks, navigating emotions and cultivating beliefs.

We are in the infancy of incorporating AI into the practice of medicine. As this technology advances, healthcare will become more accessible, timely, and cost-effective. However, the consequent challenges must be navigated, such as data privacy, ethical considerations, and workforce adaptation.

Machine Learning

Machine Learning (ML) is an AI subset that constructs decision trees to predict future outcomes. Essentially, machines 'learn' without being explicitly programmed to do so. It involves systems that simulate human intelligence by independently carrying out various tasks. ML is characterized by dynamic, iterative processes, allowing the ability to simulate human intellect. They constantly adapt to new information.

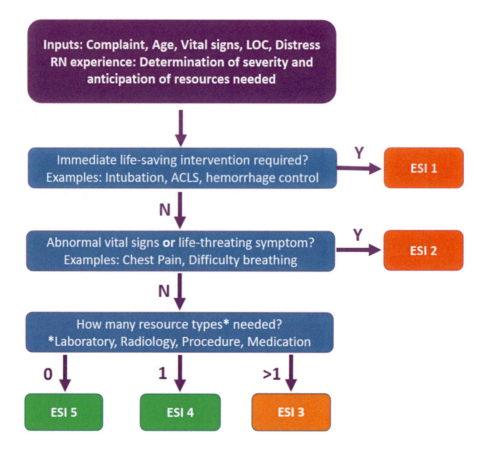

The Emergency Severity Index (ESI) is used in emergency departments to assign a triage score in a standardized manner to determine the acuity of incoming patients.

The essential elements of the ESI decision tree are shown on the opposite page. The purple box represents inputs, which are both objective (structured) and subjective (unstructured). Mednition is a company that applies ML to decipher free text in medical records and immediately assign an ESI level.

ML can entail supervised learning or unsupervised learning. *Supervised learning* uses 'training data' that contain examples of desired conclusions. For example, programs that identify cancerous cells histologically are trained on data that includes known pathology slides of cancerous cells and control slides with normal cells.

Supervised ML requires defining the goal, determining the data source, and cleaning the data. Next, a suitable machine learning model is chosen and trained. Last, results are validated, and the model is continuously adjusted.

Statistical regression uncovers associations between independent (predictors) and dependent variables (outcomes). *Simple linear regression* is utilized when a single independent variable predicts a dependent variable, producing a result. These models are simple to understand and trust, much like a spreadsheet function.

An example is the Centigrade to Fahrenheit temperature conversion. When data relationships are known, it can be relatively easy to back out the linear equation, $F° = 5/9*C° + 32$, and create a conversion algorithm.

F°	C°
-40	-40
32	0
98.6	37
212	100

Multiple linear regression is used when numerous independent variables predict a dependent variable. For example, hospital reimbursement depends on payer mix, patient volume, staffing ratios, and documentation quality. A subset of multiple linear regression is *logistic regression*, a probability of a binary output (yes or no) or ordinal output (e.g., low, medium, high) occurring by calculating odds. An example is whether a non-standard finding on a mammogram is cancer or not.

Unsupervised ML or *deep learning identifies data relationships from large datasets, such as* the *input layer*. Data processing occurs without human guidance through *hidden layers* called *artificial neural networks* (ANNs), which recognize data patterns. One pattern recognition technique is *clustering, which is* when similar data are grouped. Conversely, with *anomaly detection*, data dissimilarities are uncovered. ANN processing occurs within the "black box," whose inner workings are mysterious yet generate meaningful insights, the *output layer*.

ANNs simulate human brain function in coming to intelligent conclusions. In the context of AI, an "artificial neuron" refers to a single unit of computation within a network of neurons. This structure mimics how the human brain processes and transmits information. Neurons receive input directly from a data source or the outputs of other neurons within the network. A *weight* indicates the relative importance of the neuron's information. Also, a *bias factor* is included, allowing the neuron to adjust the weight based on data patterns. An activation function also determines if the neuron should "fire." Information from neurons that fire is forwarded to other neurons or contributes to the network's final output.

ANNs are fundamental to deep learning, a subset of machine learning, and are used in various AI applications in healthcare. Examples of deep learning in healthcare include image and speech recognition, natural language processing, and predictive analytics. A patient's medical records can be instantly compared to all medical knowledge. Identified patterns provide early disease detection and the formulation of personalized treatment plans adjusted for social determinants of health.

This figure depicts the increasing complexity of computerized decision-making from a simple decision tree to linear regression to neural networks.

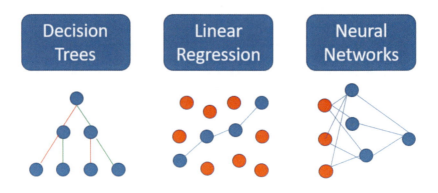

Radiomics is a technology that transforms radiographic images into quantifiable textures, colors, densities, and shapes, making expert interpretations available immediately. There will also be improved interpretation of electrocardiograms, rashes, and tissue samples.

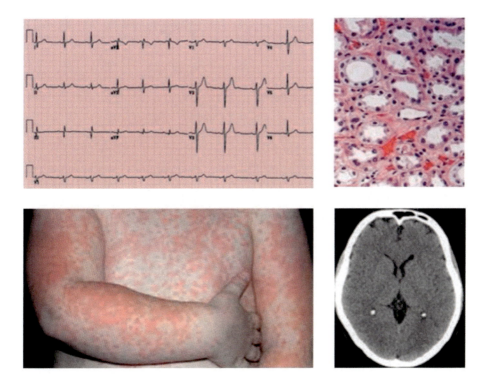

Transfer learning is a form of ML where a specific outcome is repurposed into a new model that generates different, though related, outcomes. For instance, a CT model to identify appendicitis may be repurposed to one that identifies diverticulitis. In *explainable learning*, clinicians understand the AI decision-making process, reassuring the clinician that the ML models interpret data correctly to reach reasonable conclusions. *Reinforcement learning* is a form of ML in which trial and error results in rewards or penalties. Like human psychology, reinforcement learning algorithms refine behavior based on feedback from the environment.

Four types of Deep Learning are especially applicable to healthcare professionals.

Generative AI

Generative AI is a facet of DL that uncovers data patterns and produces unique outputs, such as images and text. The ability to utilize huge data reservoirs goes beyond the limits of human intellect and imagination. [4]

Generative AI systems adapt dynamically to evolving user commands and changing input data patterns. Generative AI consumes big data sets, including every word in a patient's chart and accessible medical literature. It recommends treatment, interprets test results, augments diagnostic accuracy, guides disposition decisions, and generates billing codes. Notably, in fields like radiology and pathology, the interpretation of medical images matches or surpasses human proficiency, facilitating faster and more precise analyses. [5] Also, pharmaceutical companies are using this technology to enable the discovery of new drugs.

---

4 - https://en.wikipedia.org/wiki/Generative_artificial_intelligence
5 - https://pubs.rsna.org/doi/10.1148/radiol.223299

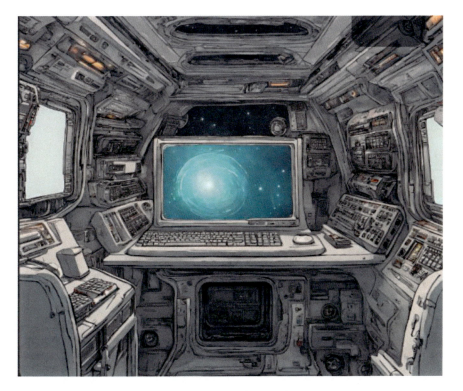

This AI-generated picture by Canva (https://canva.com) was created with the prompt, "Create a picture of a computer inside a spaceship."

Large Language Models

The large language models (LLMs) simulate human written and spoken communication in a fluid, cohesive manner, and appropriate manner. They understand language intricacies, including grammar, semantics, sentiment, and contextual nuances. An example of an *explicit statement* is, "The meeting begins at 9 am." It is simple to understand and structure. Conversely, "we've got to stop meeting like this" is an *implicit statement* requiring an understanding of semantics and context, which is accomplished by incorporating extensive textual data, including books, articles, and web content.

ChatGPT

The fourth generation of the LLM, Generative Pre-trained Transformer (GPT-4), mirrors human language. The following interchange demonstrates the ability of Chat GPT-4 to provide relevant answers to medical questions.

What are the top three causes of hemoptysis?

The top three causes of hemoptysis (coughing up blood) in adults vary based on geographical location, prevalence of certain diseases, and individual health conditions. However, in many parts of the world, the following are considered among the most common causes:

1. Bronchitis: Acute or chronic bronchitis, often due to infection or long-term irritation of the airways, can lead to inflammation and minor bleeding.

2. Pneumonia: Lung infections, whether bacterial, viral, or fungal, can cause the lung tissue to become inflamed and potentially bleed, resulting in hemoptysis.

3. Bronchiectasis: This condition involves the permanent enlargement of parts of the airways in the lungs. It leads to recurrent lung infections and can cause bleeding into the airway, resulting in hemoptysis.

Explain bronchiectasis at a fourth-grade reading level.

Imagine the tubes inside your lungs are like straws that help you breathe. Now, if those straws get damaged and become wider than they should be, it's hard for your lungs to work right. This problem is called bronchiectasis.

When the straws are too wide, germs and mucus can get stuck inside them. This can make you cough a lot, sometimes even with some goo or a little bit of blood. It's like when you're trying to drink a milkshake through a straw, but the straw is too big and gets all messy.

ChatGPT was created by OpenAI, a for-profit startup funded by Microsoft.[6] It results in instant humanlike conversation about any topic in any language around the clock. Epic Health is collaborating with OpenAI to integrate generative AI into its system. One use case is drafting responses to in-basket messages to simplify physician workflows and reduce burnout.

Machine-generated information is remarkably accurate. LLMs can pass the Attorney Bar and United States

---

6 - https://en.wikipedia.org/wiki/Large_language_model

Medical Licensing exams. With proper safeguards, such as a narrow range of questions and guardrails on patient recommendations, contact center staff can be replaced with chatbots that produce safer and more satisfying patient experiences.

Chatbots can help manage appointments, prescriptions, and referrals. Clinicians can view patient concerns, read AI-recommended actions, and appropriately respond with a summary in the medical record. Google Med-PaLM 2, an LLM chatbot that solves medical problems, is being tested at the Mayo Clinic. 7

Natural Language Processing/Speech Recognition

Natural Language Processing (NLP) enables machines to comprehend, analyze, read, and communicate by voice and text in any language. 8,9

Conversational AI improves healthcare care access by instantaneously handling nuanced conversations, adjusting to health literacy, and complying with reading-level requirements. Personalized responses can be tailored to the user's interests and preferences and even respond appropriately to sarcasm and humor.

---

7 - https://en.wikipedia.org/wiki/Natural_language_processing
8 - https://en.wikipedia.org/wiki/Predictive_analytics
9 - https://en.wikipedia.org/wiki/Natural_language_processing

Speech recognition, the technology behind robocalls, converts the spoken word to text, regardless of language or accent. Voice recognition, which identifies a voice print, can be utilized for user authentication.

NLP turns vast volumes of unstructured patient information, such as physician notes and patient-provider discussions, into structured data ready for analysis. NLP is the engine behind spam filtering, sentiment analysis, language translation, and search engines.

Dragon Ambient eXperience (DAX) Copilot by Nuance, a Microsoft subsidiary, leverages ChatGPT-4 to listen in on doctor-patient conversations, remove extraneous information, and generate concise, accurate clinical notes based on user preferences. Early adopters began using it in 2023 and found it relieved a significant burden on clinicians.

Predictive Analytics

Predictive Analytics is the DL subset used to predict unknown events. It applies statistical methods to massive datasets, deciphers intricate patterns, forecasts future outcomes, and enables informed and impactful decision-making. Moreover, it continues to learn from outcomes.

A false start with predictive analytics occurred in 2012 when IBM partnered with Memorial Sloan Kettering, a New York City-based cancer treatment and research center, to test Watson Health. The system is intended to assist oncologists in providing cutting-edge cancer treatment. Unfortunately, it did not produce relevant information, and the system was scrapped a decade later.

Recent predictive analytics technology can reliably forecast disease, accurately diagnose, and personalize patient treatment plans.

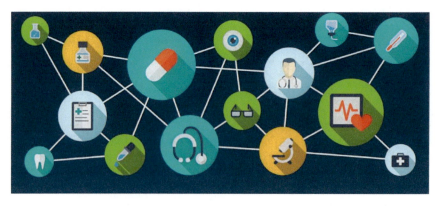

Photo credit: healthtechmagazine.com (4/17/17)

Value-Based Care

Transition from Fee-for-Service

The FFS, a traditional reimbursement system in healthcare, has been criticized for its inherent incentive structure that rewards providers for the quantity of medical services delivered rather than the quality of patient outcomes that result. [10] This model promotes overutilization and higher healthcare costs, potentially exposing patients to unnecessary risks.

The US healthcare system is transitioning from the FFS model to value-based care (VBC). In 2023, more than half of Medicare patients were enrolled in Medicare Advantage, a program that shifts reimbursement from FFS to capitation. With capitation, money is paid to a healthcare entity for service delivery based on value (quality/cost) rather than volume.

There are several cost savings models in healthcare. *Bundle payments* refer to paying hospitals and doctors a pre-negotiated amount for a complete episode of care (e.g., joint replacement). The cost of readmission and complications burdens the care providers and encourages quality improvement. With *shared savings*,

---

10 - https://en.wikipedia.org/wiki/Fee-for-service

accountable care organizations are paid like FFS, but they can share in the savings when cost is reduced. Medicare Shared Savings Plans (MSSP) include several quality measures, including disease prevention (e.g., vaccinations and screenings), disease management (e.g., complex case management), patient engagement and satisfaction (e.g., Press Ganey survey scores), and population health measures (e.g., addressing social determinants of health). Providers take on substantial risk in the *global payment* capitation model since they are paid a fixed fee for each covered patient.

Medicare Advantage and insurance products established by private insurers (e.g., Aetna, Anthem, Blue Cross, Cigna, Humana, and United Healthcare) incorporate cost incentives. Also, Amazon, CVS, Walgreens, and Walmart have entered the market and are evaluating capitated care models.

VBC represents a transformative shift in the healthcare paradigm, redirecting the focus from mere service provision to measurable patient outcomes. [11] This model encourages healthcare providers to collaborate and prioritize preventive care to achieve better patient health outcomes while optimizing resource utilization.

---

11 - https://en.wikipedia.org/wiki/Value-based_health_care

By emphasizing outcomes, VBC incentivizes healthcare providers to deliver treatments and interventions that yield tangible patient health improvements. Instead of measuring success solely by the number of services performed, the emphasis shifts to whether those services lead to better patient wellbeing and long-term health improvements.

Frameworks

In economic terms, value refers to the relationship between cost and benefits. Creating value involves optimizing resources to deliver outcomes that exceed costs and fostering success in every way, including tangible and intangible aspects.

A balanced scorecard is a crucial way to measure value. Tracking quantitative and qualitative metrics aligns business activities with strategic goals, ensuring a calculated approach to success. A framework enables organizations to assess performance comprehensively, identify areas for improvement, and make informed decisions to drive sustainable growth and enhance overall performance. It also helps understand how one value relates to another, positively or negatively. For instance, increasing staffing can reduce cost efficiency and increase patient satisfaction. Ideally, the relative value of each component in a scorecard should be measurable.

The Institute for Healthcare Improvement (IHI), a nonprofit entity founded in **1991, introduced the Triple Aim in 2006. This simple scorecard focused on quality, cost, and satisfaction.** 12 Interest in creating a more extensive and "balanced" scorecard management approach gave rise to the QUEST framework, an acronym encapsulating five facets of VBC—quality, utilization, efficiency, satisfaction, and teamwork. 13

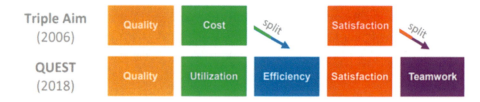

Quality

Quality in VBC refers to the measurable and consistent delivery of effective, safe, patient-centered healthcare services, optimizing outcomes and minimizing variations. It integrates evidence-based practices that yield favorable patient outcomes.

---

12 - https://www.ihi.org/Engage/Initiatives/TripleAim/Pages/default.aspx
13 - https://www.medscape.com/viewarticle/893987

Quality includes redundant safety measures that reduce the risk of morbidity and mortality. For instance, despite relaying the treatment plan after a healthcare encounter, post-encounter wellness checks can uncover missed diagnoses, rapid worsening of a disease (e.g., an asthma exacerbation), aftercare gaps (e.g., the inability to make a follow-up appointment or afford a prescription medication), and complications of a procedure.

Utilization

Utilization in VBC denotes the prudent and efficient allocation of healthcare resources, including medical interventions and services, to optimize patient outcomes while managing costs.

Improvement in test ordering requires rate measurement, identifying providers deviating significantly from the mean, and effectively coaching them.

Efficiency

Efficiency in VBC pertains to the optimal use of resources and processes so that redundancies and inefficiencies are minimized. It includes swift decision-making, parallel processing, and streamlined turnaround times.

With efficient emergency department (ED) processes, patients spend less time in the waiting room, where bad outcomes can occur when time-sensitive medical problems are not identified at triage. Also, there will be less hallway boarding waiting for an inpatient bed, which is high-risk.

Satisfaction

Satisfaction in VBC refers to fulfilling patient and provider expectations, encompassing experiences, interactions, and outcomes, contributing to overall healthcare quality.

A meta-analysis of 55 published studies validates that patient perception of high-quality care correlates tightly with evidence-based care quality. 14 Also, happy patients adhere better to aftercare plans and file fewer malpractice claims.

Teamwork

Teamwork in VBC encompasses collaborative efforts among interdisciplinary healthcare professionals, blending collective skills, knowledge, and resources to optimize patient outcomes and operational efficiency.

Stakeholders include patients, providers, payers, and system administrators. Considering all parties' objectives across the VBC spectrum cultivates an environment

---

14 - https://bmjopen.bmj.com/content/3/1/e001570

where staff experiences greater job satisfaction, fostering exceptional patient outcomes.

QUEST Dependencies

Each facet of QUEST influences the others. Optimal outcomes occur with fewer boarders (utilization), faster test results (efficiency), and more patient trust (satisfaction). Viewing quality as a dependent variable shows how it is affected by other QUEST components.

Here are examples of positive inter-relatedness using the format: Independent Variable → Dependent Variable.

Utilization → Quality: Avoiding unnecessary admissions reduces ED boarders, prevents hospital-acquired infections, reduces anxiety, and cuts superfluous tests and procedures.

Efficiency → Quality: Minimizing the time from ED arrival to departure is accomplished by shortening aspects of the patient care process. When CT scan turnaround, from the order until interpretation, is lessened, incoming patients spend less time in the waiting room, where serious problems may go unnoticed. [15]

---

15 - https://www.medpagetoday.com/opinion/second-opinions/103166

Efficiency → Satisfaction: The top factor in patient satisfaction is time to see the provider, which is minimized in highly efficient systems.

Satisfaction → Quality: A meta-analysis published in the British Medical Journal affirms that patient experience is positively associated with patient safety and clinical effectiveness across various diseases and populations. 16 The study links patient satisfaction to medication adherence and compliance with preventative care such as cancer screening and immunizations.

The QUEST framework aligns patient experience, physician expectations, system financials, and payer prerequisites, creating a strategic alignment around VBC.

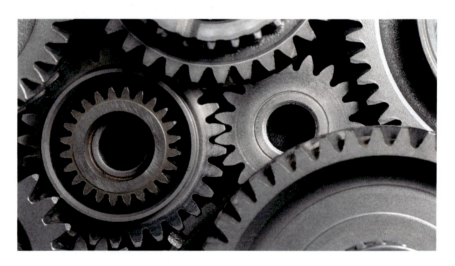

---

16 - https://bmjopen.bmj.com/content/3/1/e001570

Coupling AI and VBC

Integration

Technology integration offers a transformative solution to address some critical challenges associated with VBC, particularly the burdensome administrative tasks and complex data management requirements. As healthcare systems transition from traditional FFS models to VBC, technology becomes increasingly vital in streamlining processes and enhancing efficiency.

AI improves operational efficiency and enhances patient engagement. Patients can actively participate in their care and provide real-time health data to healthcare providers with patient portals, remote monitoring devices, and telehealth platforms. This approach aligns with VBC goals by promoting preventive measures and early interventions, ultimately leading to better patient outcomes and reduced healthcare costs.

Quality Focus

AI-driven advancements greatly enhance healthcare quality through precise diagnostics, personalized treatments, data insights, and operational streamlining. Neural networks, ML, and sophisticated speech and image processing are pivotal in achieving accurate diagnoses. Using vast datasets and cloud-based computing expedites data processing, leading to more precise diagnoses and tailored treatments.

Predictive analytics is a proactive and timely means of finding and resolving issues, enabling timely interventions. There are numerous instances of how Predictive Analytics impacts healthcare. For example, image analysis elevates diagnostic accuracy, exemplified in detecting dermatologic cancer via skin lesion images. Algorithms scrutinize electronic health records to pinpoint potential medication errors, addressing dosing, allergies, and interactions, ultimately ensuring safer patient care.

Utilization Focus

AI is especially helpful in controlling utilization. Statistical analysis detects significant provider deviations from the mean, enhancing coaching effectiveness. Alerts guide case managers in preventing specific admissions through outpatient strategies and senior care facilitation.

Safe admission avoidance is one of the most effective means of system cost control. About 30% of adult ED patients are admitted, accounting for three-quarters of all hospitalizations. Admitting versus discharging a patient is a frequent and expensive decision that emergency physicians make independently.

When hospital admissions are determined to have been avoidable, three-quarters of hospitals experience significant losses in observation status. [17] Additionally, about 40 hours of human resources are conserved when a patient is discharged.

AI includes various clinical decision support services to make informed utilization considerations.

Efficiency Focus

The increasing adoption of big data and neural networks promises to accelerate diagnoses and treatment planning. Image processing engines will expedite radiograph interpretations. AI advances healthcare efficiency by automating administrative tasks, aiding treatment planning, and streamlining processes for prompt patient care. Moreover, AI contributes to staff development by identifying knowledge gaps and refining procedural skills.

Also, leveraging historical admission trends, current occupancy rates, and seasonal infection forecasts, predictive models anticipate patient influx and tune

---

17 - https://insurancenewsnet.com/oarticle/why-patients-getting-squeezed-by-rising-number-of-hospital-observation-cases

resources for optimal efficiency. For instance, they can proactively manage staffing and bed assignments, diminishing the number of patients boarding in the ED.

An avenue for enhancing healthcare efficiency involves harnessing NLP and ML algorithms to analyze clinical documentation. These technologies precisely assign medical codes for procedures and diagnoses, expediting a traditionally time-consuming and error-prone process. This automation reduces manual workload, leading to quicker billing cycles and heightened efficiency.

Satisfaction Focus

AI enables tailored patient communication through automated engagement strategies. Data-driven approaches fuel personalized medicine by integrating demographics, history, and preferences. AI tools elevate shared decision-making and patient-centric care. Staff can gain insights into patient satisfaction and identify areas of improvement, focusing on compassion, communication, and perceived competence. Additionally, AI's efficiency enhancements afford staff more time for direct patient interaction.

Patient satisfaction experiences a boost when AI-powered chatbots offer immediate responses to inquiries about appointments, medications, and treatments. Such engagement amplifies patient communication and convenience, fostering an improved overall experience.

Teamwork Focus

AI augments teamwork by facilitating communication, automating routine tasks, fostering collaboration, aiding group decisions, monitoring burnout, boosting morale through patient feedback, and optimizing staff allocation for longevity and satisfaction.

Team collaboration platforms facilitate fluid information exchange, seamless communication, and effective collaboration across healthcare roles. By enhancing coordination and decision-making, these platforms ensure efficient patient care management by doctors, nurses, specialists, and other professionals. The result is enhanced teamwork, improved efficiency, and improved patient outcomes.

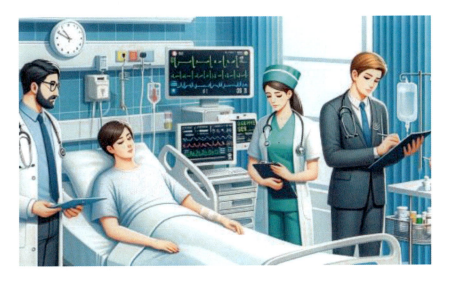

AI Across the VBC Continuum

Overview

Healthcare typically involves four interconnected phases encompassing a patient's journey, from seeking medical attention to recovery. These phases may vary in duration and complexity based on individual patient needs and the nature of the medical condition. Effective coordination and communication among healthcare professionals across these phases are essential to ensure a seamless patient experience and optimal outcomes.

Care coordination across different stages of the healthcare journey is a cornerstone of VBC. Effective communication, information sharing, and multi-disciplinary collaboration contribute to holistic patient care, minimizing redundancies and avoiding fragmented treatment approaches.

Preventing health issues is more effective and cost-efficient than treating them after they manifest. AI can identify patients at risk of returning to the ED, being readmitted to the hospital, or developing complications, thus improving population health.

There are four distinct phases in the care continuum: pre-acute, acute, post-acute, and end-of-life.

Pre-Acute Care

In the pre-acute phase, patients typically reside at home without immediate medical concerns. The primary goal is prevention. Predictive analytics allows forecasting potential health risks and intervening before an ED visit and hospitalization becomes necessary. Risk stratification is based on various factors, including demographic characteristics, past medical history, and visit patterns.

Personalized care plans are proactive measures to prevent illness and maintain good health. They contain information about vaccinations, wellness checks, cancer screenings, health education, and lifestyle recommendations.

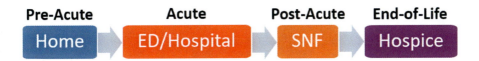

Acute Care

Acute care usually begins in the ED, where emergency physicians evaluate and treat patients with input from specialists.

Primary care physicians are overwhelmed with wellness checks and non-urgent patient issues. Most have limited capacity to address acute unscheduled patient care needs in their offices, and these cases are routinely sent to immediate care centers and EDs.

Post-Acute Care

With chronic or long-term conditions, ongoing support is necessary. This phase focuses on managing symptoms, preventing complications, and improving the patient's quality of life. It often involves lifestyle changes, regular check-ups, and continuous monitoring.

By extending care to senior living facilities, Predictive Analytics can assist in identifying patients with deteriorating health conditions. By monitoring vital signs and real-time data, algorithms can recommend timely interventions to prevent adverse outcomes and reduce hospital readmissions.

AI is increasingly used in senior living facilities to improve the quality of care, enhance safety, and provide a better overall living experience for seniors. An example in senior living facilities is remote patient monitoring and fall detection technology using cameras. [18]

---

[18] https://wires.onlinelibrary.wiley.com/doi/full/10.1002/widm.1485

End-of-Life Care

The last phase, end-of-life, is palliative and hospice care for patients with terminal or life-limiting conditions. This phase focuses on providing comfort, pain relief, and emotional support. Palliative care aims to enhance the quality of life during a patient's final days, while hospice care endeavors to keep patients comfortable and families supported during the dying process.

AI aids in end-of-life decision-making and provides logistical assistance. Data is analyzed to create personalized care plans to optimize medication dosages for symptom relief and anticipate various problems. For instance, chatbots or voice assistants navigate the complexities of palliative care, provide companionship to patients, and recommend grief support groups to families.

Of course, it is essential to maintain a balance between technological assistance and the human touch, which is crucial in end-of-life care. AI tools should complement, rather than replace, the compassionate care healthcare professionals and caregivers provide.

Case Management

Emergency Department

ED case management is well-established. In high-volume settings, they are usually stationed in the ED around the clock. They help emergency physicians and nurses coordinate patient care within a fast-paced, often chaotic, environment. They advocate for patients, ensuring their needs and preferences are considered in the treatment and care process.

ED case managers facilitate interdisciplinary communication and collaboration among healthcare professionals and family members involved in patient care. They follow up with patients the day after discharge to address concerns and ensure compliance with aftercare plans. Advanced workflow automation systems can be used to control high ED utilizers.

Inpatient

Inpatient case managers provide patients and their families with information about their conditions, treatments, and available resources, empowering them to make informed decisions.

Inpatient case managers are adept at placing patients in the correct level of care after a hospitalization, which mainly entails senior care: independent living, assisted living, and skilled nursing.

Post-Hospitalization

Case managers often address aftercare needs, particularly medication and follow-up compliance, to prevent ED visits and reduce the frequency of readmission after hospital discharge. Follow-up for complex patients may involve referrals to "transition clinics" where staff are better equipped than primary care physicians in overseeing recovery from a serious illness or injury.

Special attention is paid to patients who are medically fragile, psychiatrically impaired, substance dependent, and otherwise have barriers to obtaining primary care.

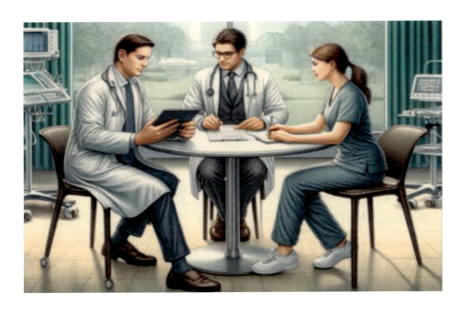

Patient-Centeredness

Personalized Care

Patient-centeredness emphasizes tailoring care to unique patient needs, preferences, and goals. This approach acknowledges that effective healthcare delivery goes beyond medical treatments, encompassing enhanced communication and active patient engagement.

Recognizing that each patient's medical history, circumstances, and goals are unique, healthcare providers design customized care plans that cater to these individual factors. Customizing a treatment plan involves considering not only medical aspects but also those socio-economic, cultural, and environmental factors that influence a patient's health journey – the social determinants of health. When healthcare providers accommodate these factors, patients are more engaged and are more likely to adhere to aftercare plans.

Ultimately, patient-centered care ensures that healthcare revolves around the patient, not vice versa. It fosters a sense of empowerment, respect, and collaboration between healthcare providers and patients.

AI creates treatment plans that integrate patient medical history and personality, prior use patterns, and medical knowledge databases to provide evidence-based treatment strategies that match an individual's needs and preferences. This approach is invaluable for complex cases where multiple factors must be considered.

AI and Empathy

While AI offers unparalleled efficiency and precision, human interactions' compassionate and empathetic qualities are irreplaceable.

Of course, excellent outcomes require making the correct diagnoses and designing effective treatment plans. Equally important is patient adherence, and this requires trust.

A critical factor in patient compliance is their trust in the care provider. Trust is derived from provider compassion, communication, and (perceived) communication, the three C's.

Compassion requires a human touch. While AI can enhance care, empathy is a uniquely human quality that technology cannot replace.

Patients trust physicians they see as competent, compassionate, and great communicators. [19] Physicians are perceived as competent when they have a professional appearance, actively listen, give the impression of being confident, and are attentive to patient needs. Compassion stems from empathy, kindness, situational mindfulness, and respect for patient autonomy.

Communication is the cornerstone of patient-centered care. Great communicators are honest and transparent. They use plain language to explain diagnoses, treatment options, and expected outcomes. They engage in open,

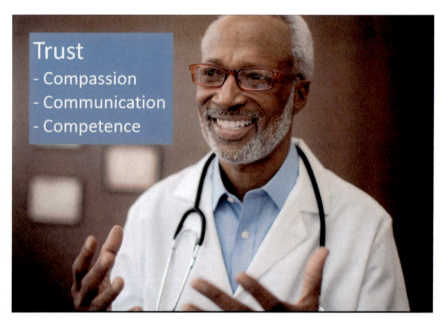

---

[19] - https://apps.aaem.org/UserFiles/file/MAAEMSeriesJanFeb19.pdf

honest, transparent, and empathetic messaging that generates a true patient-provider partnership.

AI is a supportive tool and not a replacement for human interactions. It helps healthcare professionals carve out more time to engage with patients.

Patient Activation

Patient activation relates to one's ability to follow care recommendations. Factors include a patient's knowledge level, skills, and confidence to manage their healthcare effectively. VBC models of care encourage patients to be informed decision-makers, adopt healthy behaviors, and engage with healthcare providers. Various scales determine where patients fall from being passive and disengaged to being proactive and empowered in managing their health. Higher levels of patient activation are associated with better outcomes and reduced costs.

Shared decision-making means integrating patient values and preferences into their treatment. Engaged patients experience better health outcomes and are more satisfied with their care.

Patient autonomy can be compromised by over-reliance on AI. Ensuring that patients remain at the center of healthcare decisions and have the option to choose AI-informed treatments while understanding the implications is essential.

AI Risks and Challenges

There are many risks and challenges in utilizing AI.

Users can receive inaccurate information. AI "hallucinations" are *unintentional*, errant outputs. Deepfakes are *intentional*, errant outputs used for nefarious purposes. Unfortunately, AI can make videos, images, and audio depict someone saying or doing something they never said or did.

Legal risks relate to copyright and intellectual property infringement and violations of governmental regulations regarding AI use.

AI systems derive their understanding and outputs from the data they are trained on, so a critical challenge is the phenomenon of "garbage in, garbage out." If the training data encompasses decades of content, it's likely to contain biases, inaccuracies, and insensitive perspectives related to race, religion, and other social issues, reflecting the prejudices and societal norms of earlier times.

These embedded biases can lead to AI outputs that inadvertently perpetuate stereotypes, misrepresentations, and discriminatory viewpoints, thus failing to align with contemporary efforts toward inclusivity and promoting diversity. Ensuring AI systems promote fairness and avoid perpetuating historical biases requires a concerted effort from developers, researchers, and policymakers to prioritize ethical AI development practices.

Protected Health Information (PHI) refers to sensitive and personally identifiable health-related data collected, stored, and transmitted within the healthcare ecosystem. This information includes medical records, treatment histories, payment details, and other data linked to an individual's health status.

The Health Insurance Portability and Accountability Act (HIPAA) is a comprehensive US federal law enacted to safeguard the privacy and security of PHI. HIPAA sets standards for the protection and confidential handling of PHI by healthcare providers, health plans, and business associates. It mandates practices such as obtaining patient consent for data sharing, implementing strict access controls, and notifying individuals in case of data breaches.

Maintaining healthcare data privacy and security is critical due to the sensitive nature of PHI. Unauthorized access, data breaches, and mishandling of PHI can lead to severe consequences, including identity theft, medical fraud, and compromised patient trust. These concerns necessitate robust security measures to prevent unauthorized access or hacking.

With AI, care must be taken to preserve privacy. Access to large pools of data is a setup for security breaches. Key challenges include maintaining the balance between seamless data sharing for improved patient care and maintaining stringent data privacy standards. Healthcare organizations must invest in cybersecurity measures, encryption, regular audits, and staff training to ensure compliance with HIPAA regulations and protect patient information.

Below is an example of security measures used by Auscura, a healthcare technology company that automates healthcare communication and applies smart technology to VBC use cases.

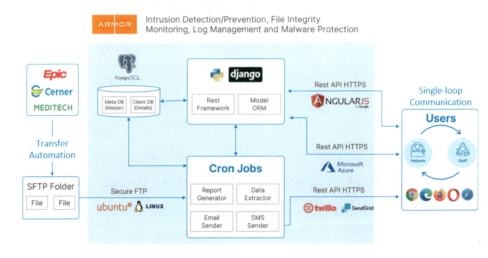

Change Management

The integration of AI can streamline routine tasks, augment diagnostic accuracy, and assist in treatment planning. Still, as with any new idea, process, system, or device, there is the challenge of user adoption. Human behavior modification is no easy feat for managers and directors. Several change management concepts are worth reviewing before any significant technology installation.

Simon Sinek: Start With Why

"Start With Why" is a concept introduced by Simon Sinek in his book and TED Talk. The core idea is that successful individuals and organizations don't just focus on what they do or how they do it; they start by clearly defining their "why" or purpose.

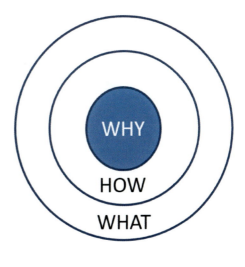

Understanding the underlying motivation behind actions and decisions creates a stronger sense of purpose and connection, both internally and externally. Beginning with the "why" helps leaders inspire staff and drive meaningful change. [20]

BJ Fogg: Change Driver

A simple change management principle is attributed to BJ Fogg, founder of the Stanford Behavior Design Lab. Fogg describes three requirements for a change: motivation, ability, and a trigger. Motivation comes from "The Why" and fundamental factors like pleasure or pain, hope or fear, and social acceptance or rejection. Ability can be impacted by time, money, physical effort, and personal convictions. Change occurs when the action line is traversed. [21]

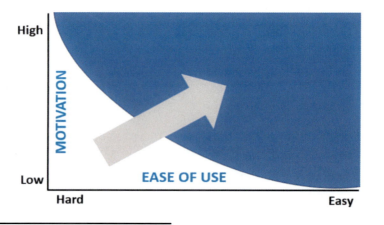

---

20 - https://www.ted.com/talks/simon_sinek_how_great_leaders_inspire_action
21 - https://web.archive.org/web/20170420144223/http://www.mebook.se/images/page_file/38/Fogg%20Behavior%20Model.pdf

Knoster's Model for Managing Change

Knoster identified five prerequisites – vision, skills, motivation, resources, and an action plan – that must be in place to change successfully. [22]

VISION	SKILLS	MOTIVATION	RESOURCES	PLAN	CHANGE
	SKILLS	MOTIVATION	RESOURCES	PLAN	CONFUSION
VISION		MOTIVATION	RESOURCES	PLAN	ANXIETY
VISION	SKILLS		RESOURCES	PLAN	RESISTANCE
VISION	SKILLS	MOTIVATION		PLAN	FRUSTRATION
VISION	SKILLS	MOTIVATION	RESOURCES		FALSE STARTS

Without clarity about what change is being planned, confusion results, causing a loss of support from stakeholders. Alleviating anxiety and apprehension requires adequate training and skill development before workflow changes. AI implementation often involves new software. There should be ample time to practice and develop confidence. Change managers must show how the change will improve the current process or outcomes. Change requires resources to be in place ahead of time, including computer hardware and support staff, to prevent frustration and apathy. A

---

22 - https://agilityportal.io/blog/knoster-model-for-change

concrete, manageable action plan prevents false starts and subsequent delays.

The Hospitalization Avoidance case study near the end of this handbook demonstrates an application of these change management principles.

Everett M Rogers: The Diffusion of Innovation

The concept of diffusion of innovation, meaning the adoption of change, was published by Everett M. Rogers in 1962. [23]

The five main characteristics of an innovation that influence adopters include (1) appreciating an advantage over the current process ("The Why"), (2) being compatible with the workflows, (3) not overly complex, (4) testing results in a positive experience, and (5) demonstrate tangible results.

Rogers defines five adopter categories, and different strategies are used to appeal to each type.

Innovators do not need to be recruited as they want to be the first to try an innovation, are willing to take risks, and often develop new ideas.

---

23 - https://en.wikipedia.org/wiki/Diffusion_of_innovations

Early Adopters are opinion leaders, usually in formal or informal leadership roles, who embrace change that makes sense.

The Early Majority accept new ideas before most, though they need definitive evidence that the innovation works, such as case studies and research.

The Late Majority are the doubters who will adopt an innovation after it has been tried and accepted by the majority and are influenced by success stories.

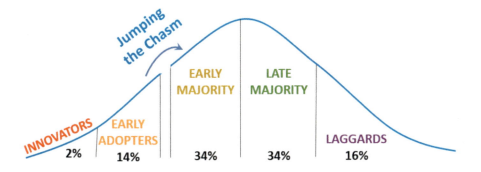

Laggards are extreme skeptics and do not need to be recruited, as they will generally succumb to peer pressure and the ramifications of job underperformance.

Rogers explains that change requires critical momentum, resulting in jumping over the chasm between Early Adopters and the Early Majority.

AI Ethics and Bias

Ensuring AI models are trained on diverse datasets is crucial to prevent biases in treatment suggestions. While AI can transform healthcare, ethical concerns center around transparency, accountability, and patient autonomy. Complex AI algorithms can foster distrust due to their 'black box' nature, making transparency essential. If not addressed, algorithm bias perpetuates inequalities in treatment recommendations, significantly affecting marginalized groups.

Accountability is challenging with AI-generated errors, requiring a balance between AI and human responsibility. There is potential for GPT models to "hallucinate" or make up answers and compellingly convey falsehoods.

Datasets must be carefully curated and cleansed of biases to ensure fair treatment. Regular audits should be performed to identify and resolve prejudicial behaviors. Collaboration among medical experts, ethicists, and communities reduces algorithmic unfairness.

Organizations must consider the impact that automation could have on displacing employees and take steps to mitigate adverse effects.

Summary

Smart technology is rapidly integrating into healthcare. While there have been excellent systems that automate workflows and use volumes of data to improve population health, there are also privacy, accuracy, and ethical risks.

Also, the transition to VBC is a fundamental shift in healthcare philosophy, changing how doctors practice, hospital staff work, and patients are treated. A practical VBC framework is QUEST, which encompasses quality, utilization, efficiency, satisfaction, and teamwork. Case management is essential to achieve VBC goals.

The US healthcare industry has surpassed manufacturing and retail to become the largest employer in the country, with every one-eighth of Americans working in this sector. There will be substantial change and associated angst, affecting many people. Healthcare leaders must understand and apply change management principles to ease staff into this new era.

Case Studies

Auscura, a healthcare technology firm, specializes in integrating intelligent solutions into VBC. Its SmartContact™ platform enables asynchronous communication among healthcare stakeholders, including patients, nurses, physicians, case managers, and patient experience leaders. This platform identifies and promptly addresses patient wellbeing and service issues following ambulatory visits.

SmartContact™ enhances VBC through workflow automation, patient engagement, and physician benchmarking, each designed to streamline operations, improve patient outcomes, and elevate the standard of care. Below are example use cases.

Hospitalization Avoidance

An effective means of healthcare cost control is safe admission avoidance. Thirty percent of adult ED patients are admitted, accounting for three-quarters of hospitalizations. The decision to admit a patient is an expensive and frequent one. [24]

One-quarter of hospital admissions are categorized as observation, typically requiring a single overnight stay.

---

24 - https://auscura.com/admits

However, three-quarters of hospital admissions retrospectively deemed avoidable were observation cases.

The SmartContact™ performance report in a high-volume, suburban ED during the fourth quarter of 2022 showed a wide range of admission rates (Adm/Tr), from 21.7% (top row) to 42.9% (second row) and a mean of 30.3% (bottom row). The red (or green) font denotes a rate higher (or lower) than one standard deviation from the mean.

RVU/h	Adm/Tr	mNPS	TAT DC	Adv Rad	Rx ATB	Rx Opiate
6.2	21.7%	55	219	40.1%	12.2%	10.7%
5.7	42.9%	73	247	59.4%	11.8%	10.7%
5.8	30.3%	54	230	42.4%	11.5%	7.6%

The highest admitter also had an excessive rate of advanced radiology (Adv Rad) testing (i.e., an order for a CT, US, or MR). He was not an outlier with the other performance metrics, including productivity (RVU/h = relative value units per hour), satisfaction (nNPS = modified net promoter score), efficiency (TAT DC = turnaround time for discharged patents), antibiotic prescribing (Rx ATB) or opiate prescribing (Rx Opiate).

The medical director's goal was to decrease admission rates safely by coaching the highest admitters. "The Why" is that US healthcare costs are unsustainable, and admission avoidance is the most significant reduction opportunity.

Using the terminology of Knoster's model, while emergency physicians are *skilled* at making disposition decisions, there is significant variability. *Motivation* includes the natural displeasure of being an outlier. The most essential *resource* is case managers finding admission alternatives. The *action plan* is monthly performance feedback.

In Fogg's model, *ease of accomplishment* is challenging as it is difficult to change the practice of those intolerant of uncertainty.

However, a remarkable change was appreciated in the physician with the highest admission rate. Key factors in his turnaround included sharing month-over-month performance, the increased frequency of consulting the ED case managers, and automated, next-day patient follow-up with SmartContact™.

He dropped to the group average, representing a cost savings of about $100,000 per year in a capitated model.

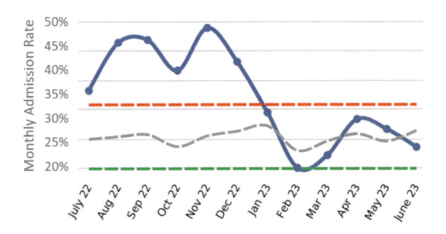

Patient wellbeing was assessed the day after discharge to screen for change-related risks using SmartContact™.

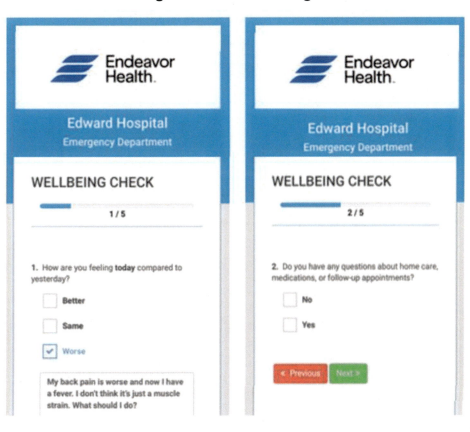

Additionally, SmartContact™ measures the rate of discharged ED patients that require admission within three calendar days of discharge and the proportion of patients reporting feeling worse.

ED Overuse Reduction

ED "superusers" sign in twelve or more times a year. This group comprises 1% of patients and 5% of all visits. High ED utilization occurs in those who are medically fragile, psychiatrically impaired, substance dependent, and with barriers to primary care.

Here is a list of the top most frequent visitors in a high-volume, suburban ED, all with upward trending. There were over 900 active superusers in the system.

Visits▼	Age/Gender	Financial Class	Latest Visit	Trend
39	70 / F	CAID ADV	07-29-23	Upward
30	50 / M	CAID ADV	07-22-23	Strongly Upward
28	65 / M	MA	08-03-23	Upward
28	73 / F	MA	08-03-23	Upward
28	39 / M	MGDCARE	07-07-23	Upward
28	48 / M	CAID ADV	08-06-23	Upward
26	67 / F	CARE	07-29-23	Upward
25	41 / M	CAID ADV	07-13-23	Upward
23	30 / M	BCBS	08-02-23	Upward

SmartContact™ automates case manager workflows, including superuser identification, care plan creation, and care network communication.

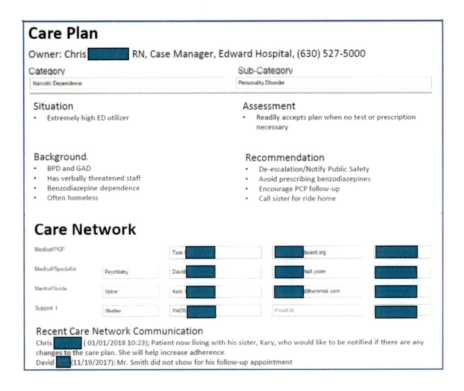

Case managers tailor interventions, engage care team members (e.g., PCP, LCSW, and POA), and meet medical needs. This tactic has been shown to cut superuser visits in half, which improves outcomes and reduces costs substantially. 25

_____

25 - https://www.auscura.com/ihi

Made in the USA
Middletown, DE
17 April 2024

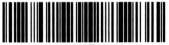